One of Jennifer's many gi|
at that very moment, and
an instant.

I love this book! In "Self Care," she continues to share that precious gift through compassion, guidance, understanding, and yes. . . nurturing. She truly believes that when you nurture your body, spirit, and soul, the rest will take care of itself, and true healing can begin.

I couldn't put it down, and you won't be able to either!

**Johnetta Alston Lake** *is the Creator, President and CEO of Inspiration Television Network*

Well before the nation (and the world) found itself engulfed by a Covid-19/ Corona Virus pandemic in the Springtime of 2020, millions of individuals had been longing for a sense of renewal, rejuvenation, and a spiritual revival, as they grasped onto various forms of nurturing themselves. Upon the sudden realization that normalcy — as all defined it — would change within a literal blink of an eye, it has become more vital than ever for even the most fervent believer to take shelter in the comforting words offered through Scripture juxtaposed with the soothing assurance of affirming testimonies.

\* \* \*

Eichelberger, an ordained minister, media practitioner, and sought-after inspirational speaker, brings us a most necessary self-care book at a most necessary time in our lives. Her third motivational read, *Self Care: The Vital Art of Nurturing You,* takes readers on a 26-chapter journey, prompted by each letter of the alphabet. The chapters are composed of conversational anecdotes, Scriptures, and a series of suggestions on how we must all take care of a most vital person: Oneself.

Now, more than ever, self-care is crucial. It is critical. *The Vital Art of Nurturing You* is a must-read. Eichelberger is also the author of the motivational titles, "Answering the Call, Discovering Your Purpose" and "The Next Level."

**Shawn Evans Mitchell** *is an award-winning veteran journalist and university professor of media arts and English composition.*

* * *

"This book enlightens the reader with both engaging anecdotes and practical advice. It's a refreshing read with real world advice worthy of every generation's time. Jennifer brings a real and yet complicated topic to the forefront."

**Shana Thornton** *is the Lead Host and Producer of Let's Talk America Radio.*

\* \* \*

In Jennifer's book, Self-Care: The Vital Art of Nurturing You, she delves into a topic that is needed now more than ever in our society. Self-care is one of the most vital natural medicines needed in our fast-paced society and Jennifer does a great job at showing us how to do just that. Her stories, insight, and in depth information and strategies helps us all learn how to practically practice self-care. Through this book you will be refreshed and inspired to do what we all need to do, take care of ourselves to be the best us! I highly recommend this book.

**Katlyn Moncrief Bryan** *is also known as "Koach Katlyn" of The Christian View.*

*Self Care: The Vital Art of Nurturing You*

Unless otherwise noted, Scriptures used are taken from the King James Version (KJV): public domain.

Scripture taken from the New King James Version®. Copyright © 1982 by Thomas Nelson. Used by permission. All rights reserved.

Scriptures marked NIV are taken from the New International Version®. Copyright© 1973, 1978, 1984, 2011 by Biblica, Inc.™ Used by permission of Zondervan

**For Information Contact:**
Jennifer Stovall Eichelberger Ministries
www.jennifereichelberger.com

ISBN for Paperback: 978-1-7349637-0-0
ISBN for eBook: 978-1-7349637-1-7

Printed in The United States of America

A Journey to Self-Care from A to Z

# SELF CARE
## *the* VITAL ART *of*
## NURTURING YOU

### A Scriptural and Practical Approach to
### Wellbeing and Wholeness

JENNIFER STOVALL EICHELBERGER

# CONTENTS

*Dedicated to my husband,*
*Dr. Herbert L. Eichelberger*
*and my sister, Karla T. Stovall*

*In Memory of...*
*Sam and Ruth Stovall*
*and my brother, Michael*

"Self care is so important. When you take time to replenish your spirit, it allows you to serve other from the overflow. You cannot serve from an empty vessel."

-Eleanor Brown

# FOREWORD

As a pastor and a psychologist who has spent his professional career seeking ways to encourage and chart paths for people to heal themselves spiritually, psychologically, and physically I have never read a more compelling book which accomplished those desired goals more than *Self Care: The Art of Nurturing You*. There are a plethora of self-help books written each year, but rarely has there been a book written with the deeply personal, transparent, compassionate feelings of Rev. Jennifer Eichelberger. This book delves into her personal journey from the pain, frustrations, disappointments, and emotional upheavals through the joys, laughter, and victories of life.

Everyone has or will encounter moments when we will come face to face with one or more of the topics outlined in this insightfully inspirational purposeful endowed epitaph. This book is certainly not a panacea for all of the emotional setbacks, past, present, or future; however, it is more than adequate to provide the reader with immediately applicable skills, knowledge, and clear directions for improving and enhancing his/her life.

After you have read this life-altering book, I can guarantee you, with ultimate assurance, that your life will be transformed for the better. You will possess the understanding as to why it is your time to finally begin to take care of yourself. Right now, I challenge you to unapologetically do something selfish. Nurture yourself into being that freshly revived person whom you have only dreamed about being, but never took time to become!

*Take care by taking self time.*

**Rev. Dr. Gerald L. Durley**
Pastor Emeritus
Providence Missionary Baptist Church

# INTRODUCTION

*Self-care is not selfish, and you can't
pour from an empty cup.*

When we log onto social media, there is no shortage of posts urging us to work harder, work faster, grind, slay, and other terms to drive us to be wealthy and successful. In this pursuit to reach the top, we overlook that health and self-care should be among our priorities. In my striving to be Superwoman, I was literally putting my health in jeopardy.

At the writing of this book, I have been working straight, without a lot of time off — a week here and there, as well as holidays. I took off as much time as was permitted, although that may not have been enough. Not to mention, while I was working, I produced a minimum of four live shows per week, without an assistant.

Yes, I have a story to tell in the hope that by sharing my

challenges and how I used these self-care tips, others will use these tools to find rest, and become renewed, restored, and revived.

There is a saying that goes something like this: "You cannot pour from an empty cup," and this is precisely where I found myself. . .empty! I had given and poured myself out so much that I started feeling depressed, cynical, and dreading going to work. I became irritable and impatient with others, soon lacking satisfaction with the job and becoming completely disillusioned. Mind you, there was a time that I absolutely enjoyed my job, but with the toxic environment that it had become, it started to take a toll on me. After experiencing all of the toxicity,

I knew I had to make a change, so I took time off to reconnect with God, family, friends, and most importantly, myself.

In the pages that follow, I will discuss how I was able to overcome burnout, with the Lord's help, and take time off for self-care. I will also talk about overcoming workplace harassment, bullying, sexism, favoritism, and nepotism; all of which can be found even in a Christian work environment.

If any of this sounds familiar to you, or if your issue looks different than mine, I believe the overarching principles and self-care tips in this book will help you. So, walk with me as I share my journey of self-care from A-Z.

# ANXIETY

"Be anxious for nothing, but in everything by prayer and supplication, with thanksgiving, let your requests be made known to God; and the peace of God, which surpasses all understanding, will guard your hearts and minds through Christ Jesus."

-Philippians 4:6-7

The word *ANXIOUS* means "experiencing worry, uneasiness, or nervousness, typically about an imminent event or something with an uncertain outcome."

It was day one of my self-care journey, and I woke up feeling nervous and anxious, but then I realized that I didn't have to go to work. I used that day to start detoxing my mind from all of the negativity that I had experienced within the last couple of years. I can tell you that this part of my self-care journey was more difficult than I had initially thought. The process of detoxing the mind can take time, as it is typically not an overnight thing.

So, it seemed that my first order of business was to quiet my anxious mind. Since I couldn't do that on my own, I had to look to someone, or something greater than myself. I found my freedom in the Word of God. Isaiah 26:3 says, "You will keep him in perfect peace, whose mind is stayed on You, because he trusts in You." And that is exactly where I started. I began to shift my focus from the problem to the solution, and over time, my anxiety began to be replaced by His peace.

Look at it like this example:

Say you have a beautiful, well-maintained yard with lush green grass adorned with some of the most gorgeous flowers one has ever seen. Then, you notice that ugly weeds have begun to pop up and invade your well-maintained landscape — what do you do? Well, most of us would pull up the weeds and put down some type of weed killer. So, do the same for your anxiety. Cut away as much negativity and worry as possible.

Worry, anxiety, stress, and negativity are the weeds that invade our garden of peace; our trust in God is the weed killer. Stop worrying and have faith and trust in God! Things will work out if you let God take control. Believe it or not, we have very little control over things.

Fortunately, for me, I did not have to take any medication. I eliminated as much 'toxicity' as I could, and I trusted God more and spent more time in prayer with Him.

SELF-CARE TIPS:

- Practice deep breathing: Inhale through your nose for about four seconds, exhale through your mouth for about eight seconds. Repeat this cycle up to four times, or until you have acquired your level of peace.

- Listen to soothing music.

- Pray and ask God for peace.

- Talk to a friend or seek professional help.

# BROKENESS

"And we know that all things work together
for good to them that love God, to them who are the called
according to his purpose."
-Romans 8:28

BROKENNESS: WE HAVE ALL EXPERIENCED IT. SO, WHAT IS it? I am not necessarily talking about just a broken heart, but this degree of brokenness also includes a broken spirit.

Is something perplexing you? Did someone break your heart? Is something diverting your attention from your purpose, calling, or ministry? Are you discouraged? Are you feeling frustrated, downtrodden, hopeless, helpless, and empty? Are you facing a trial that seems impossible to bear? Hang in there; we are going somewhere.

I experienced brokenness at one particular point in my life. I had a wonderful job that I thoroughly enjoyed. It warranted me the opportunity to meet people from all over the world, plus I enjoyed the creative aspect. There was one thing missing... I never felt appreciated by my immediate administrator. As hard as I worked, putting my best foot forward daily, not once did this person thank me for a job well done. Sure, expressions of gratitude were given at Christmas, but that was to the whole staff; other than that, nothing but complaints.

We all like to know that we are doing a good job, and it is good to hear that from time to time. However, when you continually hear negative feedback on trivial things, it will start to work on you inside. You begin to feel useless, and your self-worth will suffer. Still, we must remember that we are doing a work unto the Lord and not man. The job does not supply all of my needs; it is God who does. You see, our job is a means to an end, not our complete source or resource. God is our supplier, not our jobs, mates, or other things we may deem as the source — it is God.

It was not the same because somehow, I felt like I was not contributing — strange, but that is how I felt at that time. Anyway, I was broken because I had placed my faith in things and not in God. I learned that anything that gets in the way of our walk with God would, sooner or later, be removed.

As part of our Christian walk, we will go through seasons of brokenness in order for God to make us fit for His kingdom purpose. However, brokenness is not a weakness; it merely means we are wholly dependent on God. Let me give you a quick analogy: In Kintsugi, (the Japanese artistic process of repairing 'broken' pottery with liquid gold) the vessel is strengthened, and the broken area becomes stronger than the whole portion.

> And He said to me, 'My grace is sufficient for you, for My strength is made perfect in weakness.' Therefore, most gladly I will rather boast in my infirmities, that the power of Christ may rest upon me. Therefore, I take pleasure in infirmities, in reproaches, in needs, in persecutions, in distresses, for Christ's sake. For when I am weak, then I am strong.

> -2 Corinthians 12:9-10

Our Father will allow brokenness in our lives, whether we want to go through this season or not, it is part of the process that will ultimately make us stronger and propel us to fill our God-given purpose.

Also, brokenness is God's way of dealing with our self-reliance and self-dependency — in other words, *pride*. When we give our lives to Christ, we should submit every area of our lives to His will; then He uses our trials and tribulations to lead us to the point of total surrender. Brokenness is not punishment; however, God does chastise us for our sins and wrongdoing, but for the record, *brokenness* is not necessarily punishment. It is, however, to bring out the best in us. When we are broken, we are closer to the Father. Psalm 34:18 says, "The Lord is near to those who have a broken heart, And saves such as have a contrite spirit." That is what I meant earlier when I said brokenness is not such a bad thing after all.

There are many Old and New Testament saints that went through a season of brokenness . . . Moses, Job, David, and Paul, just to name a few, and they did great and mighty things for the Lord. We, too, can do great and mighty things, if we choose not to resist this process.

Submit your will to God's perfect will, because there are consequences to entertaining brokenness:

- It will impede our relationship with God.
- It delays the fulfillment of God's will in our lives; it will prevent us from experiencing His blessings and future rewards.
- It can limit what God can do through our gifts and talents.
- It can cause unnecessary delay.

SELF-CARE TIPS:

Meditate on the following:

- *If you are dealing with pride, exchange that for humility.* "Therefore, humble yourselves under the mighty hand of God, that He may exalt you in due time." -1 Peter 5:6

- *If you are dealing with impatience, exchange it for patience.* "But let patience have its perfect work, that you may be perfect and complete, lacking nothing." -James 1:4

- *If you are disobedient from time to time, exchange that for obedience.* "If you are willing and obedient, you shall eat the good of the land." -Isaiah 1:19

- *If you are allowing anything before your relationship with God,* remember He is the great I AM, and we should have no other gods before Him.

## CELEBRATE YOURSELF

"I will praise You, for I am fearfully
and wonderfully made; Marvelous are Your works,
and that my soul knows very well."
-Psalm 139:14

THAT IS CORRECT; YOU READ IT RIGHT! CELEBRATE
yourself. The enemy uses many tricks and devices to disrupt our
Christian walk. Feelings of unworthiness, low self-esteem, and
self-hatred are all part of the devil's bag of tricks and schemes.
But, do you know what? God has created us for greatness. Don't
let anybody tell you that you are not good enough, pretty
enough, smart enough, or rich enough for God's blessings.

We even sometimes feel so bad about ourselves that when
God pours out a blessing for us, we question the good things in
life. We must stop thinking like that. If God has blessed you
with something, then thank Him for it. It is a gift from Him.

Don't sit around and let someone talk you out of your blessings. Women tend to put others first; such as working on projects without asking for help, taking our mental and physical health for granted, or not prioritizing our needs.

We sit around and say to ourselves *'no one will ever want me because I am too tall, too short, too fat, too old, too young, too dark, too light, or too this or too that'*. You see, low self-esteem can cause us to remain in toxic relationships, stay on jobs that we hate, and stop us from living out our dreams, or fulfilling our destiny. Please be satisfied with yourself. Celebrate yourself. If you are not happy with your looks, make the appropriate change for yourself, not others. Remember, God looks at the heart.

Referring to the section on brokenness, somehow, I was waiting to be validated by my superior — when I actually should have been concerned about what God said about me. As long as you know that you are doing a good job, doing the best you can, the rest doesn't matter. Stop waiting to be validated by someone else. Instead, look at what God says about you.

1 Peter 2:9 states, "But you are a chosen generation, a royal priesthood, a holy nation, His own special people, that you may proclaim the praises of Him who called you out of darkness into His marvelous light." You are royalty — which means you are a prince or princess, or a king or queen.

Psalm 139:14 says, "I will praise You, for I am fearfully and wonderfully made; Marvelous are Your works, And that my soul knows very well." The keywords in this passage of Scripture are 'fearfully and wonderfully made'. God took time and care to make each one of us according to His image.

SELF-CARE TIPS:

- Travel.

- Schedule a few visits to a health and beauty spa and allow someone else to pamper you; to include pedicure, manicure, and makeover.

- Embrace your body, as long as you are healthy and satisfied with yourself. Eat healthily and drink plenty of water.

- Exercise: e.g. walk, yoga, or Pilates.

- Never forget what God says about you. Remember, we are the apple of His eye!

# DISTRACTIONS

"Let your eyes look straight ahead,
and your eyelids look right before you. Ponder the path of your
feet, and let all your ways be established. Do not turn to the
right or the left; remove your foot from evil."
-Proverbs 4:25-27

DISTRACTIONS CAN SHOW UP IN VARIOUS FORMS: AN
unexpected illness, an emergency of some kind, demands of a
job, business, ministry, bills, a computer virus, a stalled-out car,
or a flat tire. Even relationships can distract us from our God-
given goals. Not to mention, the social networking of late, too,
can be a huge distraction for many if not prioritized, or used
with a purpose in mind. So, be careful of those who demand
your attention.

We live in an ever-changing world that demands much of
our attention, and if we are not focused, it will throw us off-

track. We somehow feel that we must participate in all that is coming our way. We think we 'need' to attend this conference, that function or event; this awards show, that program, and all of the other functions that are going on.

We have taken on a 'superhero' mentality, thinking we are the be-all and can-do-all, and if we are not careful, we will either end up burnt-out, or not accomplishing anything at all. Hence, our focus is diverted from what is truly important. Recognize that the distraction is something that divides your attention or blocks your concentration. Yes, situations in life (or curveballs) will happen, but give it the proper time and attention and move on. Don't dwell on it. Fix it, repair, discard it and move on.

Yes, people will come our way to garner attention, have their needs met, and fulfill personal agendas. In that case, exercise discernment; if it is not God-ordained, if it is not propelling you to Christ or enhancing your God-given purpose, then remove yourself from that distraction.


## SELF-CARE TIPS:


- *Focus on Jesus!* In Matthew 14:28-31, we are
  reminded to keep our eyes on Jesus. Peter was
  walking on water toward Jesus, but when the
  distraction came (in this case, the wind), he focused
  on the distraction rather than Jesus and began to
  sink — but thank God, Jesus was there to catch him.

So, whatever you are facing, keep your eyes on Jesus!

- *Press on!* Philippians 3:13-13 reminds us to "Press toward the mark for the prize of God's high calling in Christ Jesus." Whatever assignment you have from God, be it to write a book, start a business, start a ministry, evangelize to the nations, or whatever God has called you to do, keep that in the forefront of your mind and press on!

- *Know that you are worthy of His calling!* When we read 2 Thessalonians 1:11-12, we are reminded that God has counted us worthy of His calling. As I stated earlier, many distractions can be fixed, repaired, or discarded, but when it comes to people, remember God has called you for that assignment, and let nothing become a distraction. Yes, we all need each other, but we don't want to block each other's concentration.

- Prioritize and be intentional.

# ENDURANCE

"Therefore, having been justified by faith, we have peace with God through our Lord Jesus Christ, through whom also we have access by faith into this grace in which we stand, and rejoice in the hope of the glory of God. Not only that, but we also glory in tribulations, knowing that tribulation produces perseverance; and perseverance, character; and hope. Now hope does not disappoint, because the love of God has been poured out in our hearts by the Holy Spirit who was given to us."

-Romans 5:1-5

ENDURANCE IS A COMPONENT OF THE FRUIT OF THE SPIRIT. It is the quality of longsuffering, which includes patience, steadfastness, restraint, and self-control. Endurance is often used interchangeably with patience. The funny thing about this word is, if you look up endurance, it mentions patience and vice versa.

Webster's Dictionary defines patience as "endurance of pain or provocation without complaint", and the "power to wait calmly and to preserve." My definition of endurance and patience is having to wait for something, even though I don't want to. I want it, and I want it right now!

Why? Wait? What?

*Wait* is a dirty word in today's society! But as Christians, we are all enduring or waiting for something. The Bible clearly states in Hebrew 10:36 that "...you have need of endurance, so that after you have done the will of God, you may receive the promise." If we want the promises of God, we must endure and be patient. As mentioned earlier, we are all waiting on God for something.

You may be waiting on God for a job, healing (physical, mental or spiritual), a new home, finances, or something else that you have asked God for — we must endure. Some of you reading this may be waiting to conceive, to have your first child, and enduring all that is involved with that process; yet, others are enduring trials in their relationship.

In times past, I suffered and endured many things, and God came through for me. So, from personal experience, I know that God will answer your prayer. In the meantime, here in the following are some steps on what to do while you are enduring. *Keep your hope in the Lord!*

## SELF- CARE TIPS

- *Recognize that God has the perfect plan for your life.* "For I know the thoughts that I think toward you, says the Lord, thoughts of peace and not of evil, to give you a future and a hope." - Jeremiah 29:11

- *Recognize that God is always with you.* "Let your conduct be without covetousness; be content with such things as you have. For He Himself has said, 'I will never leave you nor forsake you.'" -Hebrews 13:5

- *Recognize and wait on God's perfect timing.*

- *Place all of your trust in God.* "Trust in the Lord with all your heart, and lean not on your own understanding; In all your ways acknowledge Him, And He shall direct your paths." -Proverbs 3:5-6

# FEAR

"When anxiety was great within me,
your consolation brought joy to my soul."
-Psalm 94:19

I HAVE TO TAKE A DEEP BREATH ON THIS ONE. NO, I AM NOT having an anxiety attack; that is over and done with, but now, we are dealing with fear — an emotion that we can and must do without. Fear is described as bondage, torment, and a snare. It can stop you dead in your tracks and, if left unchecked, it will paralyze you, hinder you and your prayers, limit your faith, and distort your vision. Fear can stop you from answering your call, discovering your purpose, and keep you from moving to the next level. In the end, fear will keep you from being all that God has called you to be.

Many people are feeling helpless and hopeless because of fear. Fear takes on many forms: fear of failure, fear of success, fear of the future, fear of death, and even life after death. Well, God did not intend for us to operate like that. The media has us fearful of the economy, harmful products or services, food, medicines, cars, weather, wars, conflict, crime, and most recently, the COVID-19 pandemic... and the list goes on.

I, too, had to overcome fear. Some years ago, early in the ministry, I was asked to do the opening praying for a church program. I was so fearful and nervous that I had myself so worked up that day, that I literally became physically ill and had to call in to say that I would not be able to do the prayer. Then, when I wrote my first book, one of my girlfriends said, "You know you will be called on to speak because people are going to want to meet the author." Still, it took time, prayer, and practice to overcome this.

You can also overcome whatever fear you have. Just remember this . . . 2 Timothy 1:7 says, "For God hath not given us the spirit of fear; but of power, and of love, and of a sound mind." When you are preparing to do something, like speaking in public, a job interview, or whatever you are fearful of, repeat that Scripture over and over as many times as necessary until fear dissipates. Also, one way to overcome a fear is to do whatever you are fearful of.

Well, look at me now. God has opened many doors for me to speak at conferences, on the radio, and television interviews. Do I still get nervous? Sure, I do, but I am not going to allow fear to dictate my life, and neither should you. President Franklin Roosevelt, in his 1933 Inaugural Address, made mention that "There is nothing to fear but fear itself."

As Christians, we absolutely cannot operate in fear. If we are operating in fear, then we are not operating in faith. It is just that simple. So, let's replace that fear with faith. When fear tries to come upon you, put your faith into operation!

*Do not allow fear and anxiety to control your life.*

SELF-CARE TIPS:

- *We do not need to fear anyone or anything.* Why? Because Psalm 27:1 tells us that "The Lord is my light and my salvation; whom shall I fear? The Lord is the strength of my life; of whom shall I be afraid?"

- Visualize yourself unafraid.

- Confront your fears with faith.

- Most of us are familiar with the Psalm 23, with emphasis on verse 4, "Yea, though I walk through the valley of the shadow of death, I will fear no evil: for thou art with me; thy rod and thy staff, they comfort me."

- Live in the moment!

25

# GRATITUDE

"I will praise the Lord according to
His righteousness, and will sing praise
to the name of the Lord Most High."
-Psalm 7:17

GRATITUDE IS A WORD THAT EXPRESSES THANKS AND
praise to God; it is an essential component of self-care. No
matter how stressful your life may be, when you take a moment
to count your blessings, it will completely change your life.
When you are grateful for the things you have, no matter how
small, that thing will begin to increase. There is always
something to be grateful for: life, health, strength, food, clothing,
and shelter, to name a few.

A spiritual father and close friend of our family gave me
some practical advice on how to handle the problematic
workplace environment that I was experiencing. He said,

"When you wake up in the morning, give God thanks, and continue to trust Him." That is exactly what I focused on; being intentionally thankful, and of course, trusting God.

Gratitude shows God that no matter how challenging life can be, you are thankful, nonetheless. Think of it this way . . . when you give someone a gift or do something nice for them, basically, all you want in return is a *thank you* — an act of appreciation. God is the same; He simply wants our gratitude.

Be intentional when being grateful. Be grateful for your family and relationships. Be grateful for your employment, your business, and your finances. Be grateful for clean water, family, joy, peace — and anything else you can think of — just be grateful. Even if things are not where you want them to be, continue to be thankful.


SELF-CARE TIPS:


- Keep a gratitude journal. Each day, write down ten to fifteen things you are grateful for.

- Handwrite a *thank you* note and send it to someone.

- Perform random acts of kindness.

- Meditate on Palms 136.

# HEALTH AND HEALING

"Beloved, I wish above all things that
thou mayest prosper and be in health, even
as thy soul prospereth."
-3 John 2

SEVERAL YEARS AGO, I WENT IN FOR A ROUTINE PHYSICAL
examination. A few days later, I received a call asking me to
return to their office, as soon as possible, because some of my
test results were abnormal and I could have a severe ailment.
Now, I have been transparent with you, thus far, in this book,
and I will continue to do so.

So, what did I do? I panicked! Yes, I did. I panicked. I had
no clue what I was going to face when I arrived at the doctor's
office. The question now was, what was I going to do?
Remember, the name of this book is "Self-care".

As I have stated earlier, God has equipped us for anything

that comes our way. This means that I can handle this, too, with the help of the Lord. But first, let me say this . . . the abnormal test result was that of high blood pressure, borderline diabetes, elevated cholesterol, and impending kidney issues. Hold up, wait a minute. Me?

However, the news wasn't too bad, except for the kidney issues, which is a big concern since kidney disease runs on both sides of my family. So, as I was sitting in the doctor's office, my next question was, "What do I do?" The doctor said, "Here is your action plan: eat properly, exercise, and lose weight." I mentally added prayer to the list and said, "I can handle that." And that is exactly what I did. I prayed and called on everyone that I thought could get a prayer through.

Each time I thought about it, I would lay my hands on my back and pray for my kidneys. Funny thing, I later found out that the kidneys are not really in your back, but more on the side — anyway, that is what I did. And, the kidney ailment had been healed by the time I got to the nephrologist (kidney specialist).

But again, I had to do my part with diet, exercise, and of course, prayer. Five months later, I went for a follow-up appointment and had lost about twenty pounds; and my test results were better. Just recently, I went for a checkup, and the doctors said, "Whatever you are doing, keep it up."

My aim is not to make anyone feel bad about their weight, but statistics show Americans continue to be overweight, and suffering from preventable diseases. It does not have to be like that. Listen to your health care professional, listen to me; you can turn those things around. I know we think our weight is cool, "we big girls and big boys look good," and that might be true, but what about your health?

If you are overweight and healthy, that is fine, but sooner or later, that weight may catch up with you, in more ways than one. I have lost a total of fifty pounds, I run or jog up to about four to five miles at least six times a week, and the benefits are worth it. Not only do I look good, but I feel good, and I no longer have the ailments that I mentioned earlier.

SELF-CARE TIPS:

- First of all, if you are sick, let go of all un-forgiveness, resentment, anger, guilt, shame, jealousy, and envy toward anyone. Those things are the works of the flesh and will rot your bones (Proverbs 14:30). Let it go, now. Remember, your body is the temple of the Holy Spirit, and you want your healing process to begin this very moment.

- Second, watch how you treat your body. Become more aware of your diet, exercise, and proper rest. Think Godly thoughts, eat healthy food, drink plenty of water, and exercise regularly. Reduce the dangerous belly fat. Everyone is not going to be a size twelve, but that doesn't mean you have to be a twenty plus-size either. I love you and care enough to tell you this. Please listen!

- Third, stay in the Lord's presence because this is where you will gain your strength and healing. Set aside time every day to talk to God.

- Fourth, saturate your spirit with healing scriptures that are found throughout the Bible.

- And finally, avoid stress and stressful situations. Watch what you say, speak with love and kindness. For every negative word you speak, it takes three positives things to counter the negative word.

# INTEGRITY

"Providing honorable things, not only in the sight
of the Lord, but also in the sight of men."
-2 Corinthians 8:21

WEBSTER'S DICTIONARY DEFINES *INTEGRITY* AS:

1: firm adherence to a code of especially *moral* or artistic
values: *incorruptibility* 2: an unimpaired condition:
*soundness* 3: the quality or state of being complete or
undivided: *completeness*

Some even define integrity as a reputation, but it is far
deeper than that. Yes, it is quality of *character*; however, it is also
what's on the inside that exudes on the outside. Integrity is the
whole makeup of a person. We should all strive to live according

to the biblical model that God has set for us, but we often tend to fall short of that.

As I think about when I was a single Christian woman, there had been times when I did not live up to the standard that God had set for me. By compromising, I would often end up being hurt and disappointed, while experiencing guilt and shame. So, rather than go through that, I decided to remain celibate (with the help of my Lord and Savior) until I married. Was it easy? The answer to that is no. But, was it worth it? Absolutely! Because, now I am married to a wonderful man who God hand-picked just for me. As a minister of the gospel, I must do what I can to live up to God's standard.

Now, some of you may be struggling with various issues that may cause you to compromise your integrity, but whatever it is, confess it, repent, and move forward. Integrity should cause all of us to do the will of God and walk in His ways.

There are way too many headline stories about people in a high position, be it political leaders or spiritual leaders. They show that their integrity is in stark contrast with the position. This is going to sound preachy, but if you have a position that God has called you to, please do the best you can to live up to that standard.

Many often talk about raising the standards. Well, the standard has already been set. We just need to live up to it! The world is looking for leaders to mess up, and unfortunately, many of us mess up royally. Whenever a situation comes up, take the high road, regardless of whatever others may say.

We are living in a time when right seems wrong and wrong

34

seems right. Doing things the right way will ultimately pay off. *Integrity is essential for self-care.*

SELF-CARE TIPS:

- Live a life of integrity will free you from shame and guilt. "But we have renounced the hidden things of shame, not walking in craftiness nor handling the word of God deceitfully, but by manifestation of the truth commending ourselves to every man's conscience in the sight of God." -2 Cor. 4:2

- Limit association with evil doers—unless you are witnessing to them about Christ.

- Be determined to live an honorable life. "Having your conduct honorable among the Gentiles, that when they speak against you as evildoers, they may, by your good works which they observe, glorify God in the day of visitation." -1 Peter 2:12

- Speak well of others and fact-check information before sharing or posting on social media. Nip gossip in the bud.

- Show kindness and respect to others.

# JEALOUSY TO ENVY TO JOY

"You will show me the path of life; In
Your presence is fullness of joy; At Your right hand
are pleasures forevermore."
-Psalm 16:11

JEALOUSY AND ENVY ARE SO CLOSELY RELATED THAT IT IS
challenging to distinguish between the two. As I researched the
definition for the word jealous, I was somewhat surprised at
what I discovered. But I think I found a term that I am
comfortable with for this particular section of the book.

An online Yahoo dictionary defines *jealous* as:

1: Fearful or wary of being supplanted; apprehensive of
losing affection or position.

JENNIFER STOVALL EICHELBERGER

2: Resentful or bitter in rivalry; envious: *jealous of the success of others.*

3: Inclined to suspect rivalry.

4. Having to do with or arising from feelings of envy, apprehension, or bitterness: *jealous thoughts.*

For this piece, I will focus on this definition: resentment or bitterness in rivalry towards others' success. If we are truly honest about it, we have probably been jealous of someone at some point in time. I know I have. I would find myself saying things like 'how did she get that car?' 'How did she get that promotion?' 'She must spend all of her money on clothes!' 'How did she get him?' 'She just went on another vacation.' 'How many pairs of shoes does she think she needs?'

I know it sounds immature and superficial, but that is where I was at in that time of my life.

Not to mention the jealousy that goes on in church: 'she or he is singing my song.' 'How did they get to preach?' I must add that, unfortunately, jealousy in the church can seem worse than in the world. If we are not careful, jealousy will escalate into envy, which is *to feel resentful and unhappy because someone else has, or has achieved, what one wishes to possess or achieve.* If left unchecked, this can devolve into bitterness or covetousness, and in the worst case, murder.

In short, when we are jealous or envious of someone or

something, in essence, we are telling God that He doesn't know what He is doing.

I know that is "tight, but it is right." Unfortunately, I have been on the receiving end of someone being envious and jealous of me. Let me tell you; it was an ugly situation.

Our society is built on getting more and more at any cost. What others have has become such a pervasive aspect of our culture that the media thrives on it — consistently showing us what others have materially, whether they received it honestly or not. Know that what God has for you is for you.

SELF-CARE TIPS:

- Ask God to deliver you from that spirit of envy and jealousy. He will do it; God delivered me from it.

- Trust that God will supply all of your needs in His time and His method.

- God is no respecter of persons; "if you are willing and obedient, you can eat the good of the land." - Isaiah 1:19

- Set your own goals and level of success. You may not have been called to pastor a megachurch, you may not be qualified to head a department just yet, or you may not be ready for some of the things you desire at this time.

- Do what you can do to prepare for your blessing; go back to school, research, and study the habits of successful Christian individuals. Instead of being jealous or envious of someone successful, remember that we don't know what seeds they have sown, and it just might be their time to be blessed in that area.

- Be joyful of others' achievements. Be joyful, regardless of what your situation may be. Have the joy that is not based on temporary pleasure, but God's blessings. Be thankful for what God has given you — health, family, friends, food, clothes and shelter. In short, work on a better you.

# KEEPER

"The LORD *is* your keeper..."
-Psalms 121:5

SOME WORDS THAT ARE SYNONYMOUS WITH "KEEPER" ARE custodians, protectors, shields, and defenders, which is exactly what God will do for us; all of that and so much more. In this chapter, 'keeper' is a powerful portion of my testimony because I must talk about the extraordinary things that God has done for me; and how He 'kept' me during some difficult situations.

I mentioned earlier that I had been celibate for some years before getting married to my wonderful husband. And of course, during that time, there were some moments when I wanted to give in and compromise my integrity and Christian walk, but my Lord and Savior stepped in and kept me, protecting me from a lifetime of hurt and pain. He kept me during all of the crises and calamities that I have faced in life.

There is a familiar poem entitled, "Footprints in the Sand" by Mary Stevenson, where the writer refers to times in her life when she notices two sets of footprints and other times when there was only one set. She soon realizes that the one set was when Jesus was carrying her during a difficult time. That poem is an excellent example of how God is a keeper, even when we think He is not there for us.

There have been times that I felt like I was going to lose my mind, but God kept me; if you put your trust in Him, He will also keep you. I know God has kept you and protected you from dangers, seen and unseen — that car accident, that life-threatening disease, that suspicious situation, etc. Whatever you are faced with, remember, God is a keeper. The entire chapter of Psalms 121 sums it all up! He is our keeper!

SELF-CARE TIPS:

- God will keep (shield) us from the wiles and tricks of the enemy — He is our shield. "But thou, O LORD, art a shield for me; my glory, and the lifter up of mine head." -Psalm 3:3

- He is our rock. "The LORD is my rock, and my fortress, and my deliverer; my God, my strength, in whom I will trust; my buckler, and the horn of my salvation, and my high tower." -Psalms 18:2

- He is our protector. "But let all those that put their trust in thee rejoice: let them ever shout for joy, because thou defendest them: let them also that love thy name be joyful in thee." -Psalms 5:11

- Relax, breathe, and rest, knowing that God has everything in control.

# LIFE

"The thief does not come except to steal, and to kill,
and to destroy. I have come that they may have life,
and that they may have *it* more abundantly."
-John 10:10

LIFE IS A CHARACTERISTIC STATE, OR MODE, OF LIVING; THE
course of human events and activities that are different for all of
us, and this book are about facing all kinds of issues in Life.

Oh yes, we all have the basic needs in life, generally known
as Maslow's hierarchy of needs — physiological, safety,
love/belonging, esteem, and self-actualization, but we still have
individual things that make us unique. However, without God
providing the basic need for us, it goes without saying that we
would not have life.

As we go about this particular state, or mode, of living, I
have seen many people that go from day to day without any real

purpose or plan. By failing to make decisions, they demonstrate an attitude of "let the chips fall where they may." This is a fatalistic approach to life.

When one fails to plan or make decisions, they are simply giving their power over to others to make those decisions for them — except, of course, when you give your life to Christ as your personal Savior — because not only does He give us life, He offers abundant life. However, the key to this abundant life is the willingness to allow Him to lead, and being obedient to follow His plan for our life.

It is important to note that what may be successful to one, may not be successful for another. I realized that if we are not facing adversity, we will not be able to live life to the fullest. Let me explain . . . in my life, as a television producer and minister, I have met many people from all walks of life. I have met rich, poor, successful, and those that settle for mediocrity. I have met corporate people and those that are hourly wage earners. I have met world travelers and those who have never traveled beyond their hometown, let alone their state. I have met the movers and shakers and the fewer actives. I have met those that have a perfectly fit body and those that do not exercise at all. And, I have met those that multi-task, and those who don't task at all.

The point I am making here is that I have met people on both sides of the spectrum. All of these people are living, but not all are living life to the fullest (abundant life). God created us to live a life of abundance, but the enemy came to kill, steal, and destroy that plan. Let me explain further. Those considered to be at the top of their "game" are overcomers and will push beyond their issues of life. Yes, disappointments will come, discouragement will come, fear will rear its ugly head, setbacks and rejections will come. But you know what? That is all part of life. When these things happen, that does not mean to stop living by crawling into the proverbial hole.

1 Peter 4:12 says, "Beloved, think it not strange concerning the fiery trial which is to try you, as though some strange thing happened unto you." This Scripture explains what I am trying to say. Things will happen, if you are living the life of a Godly Christian, and especially if you are living the life that God has for you. So, live! And live life to the fullest.

It is a gift from God!

## SELF-CARE TIPS:

- Live the life of abundance that God has for you.

- Set your goals, organize, and prioritize. Defy the odds, because you can do all things through Christ. Find your level of success and live it!

- Turn your stumbling blocks into stepping stones.

- Practice deep breathing and meditation.

# MATERIAL POSSESSION

"No one can serve two masters; for either
he will hate the one and love the other, or else
he will be loyal to the one and despise the other.
You cannot serve God and mammon."
-Matthew 6:24

MATERIALISM HAS BECOME A PART OF OUR CULTURE, especially American culture. We now live in a time when the attitude is "he [or she] that has the most toys wins." My question to that statement is, *wins what?*

Materialism can be defined as someone with a great desire for material possessions, with little thought to their spirituality — admittedly, that is a little extreme; however, in pursuit of the American dream is what it almost boils down to. If we are not careful, we can all get caught in that.

There was a time when I had gotten caught up. About

twenty years ago, when living in certain parts of the country, especially the large metropolitan cities, I was introduced to an attorney who was from a prominent family in the D.C. area. I was "warned" about his family — that I should dress a certain way, drive a specific car, live in a particular area — you get my drift. Keep in mind, I was a lot younger then, but I found myself living way beyond my means to fit in with his family and friends... and for what?

I remember going to affairs with them (and yes, I was dressed to impress), but when I would come home, I would look at myself and think, *girl, none of this stuff is paid for.* I mean nothing, from the shoes to the car to the furniture, all because I was caught up in acquiring material possessions to please someone else. How crazy is that?

In that same way, many of us get caught up in materialism. Thank God I have been delivered from that, and I am debt-free! God wants His children to prosper. He delights in the prosperity of His children; however, we must not forget that He is the source of our blessings. True prosperity includes total well-being: health, good relationships with family and friends, peace, and a purpose-filled, joyful life. Still, we often feel that the more we have, the better off we are, and in some cases, we end up feeling emptier. Sometimes, we put so much emphasis on the outside that we end up in debt, which in some cases, leads to financial disaster.

At times, we rely on our material possession and allow it to identify us and make us feel secure. I am not much different from the next person; I like high-end things. However, now I use wisdom and knowledge when making purchases. Still, too many of us are caught up in what a person drives instead of what drives the person.

## WHY DO WE WANT TO ACCUMULATE MORE?

Because we tend to think that money and material possessions are the answer. No, God is the answer to all of our problems. Now, remember, God wants us to prosper; He wants us to have nice things. . .he just doesn't want things to have us. Ultimately, we should put our trust in God and accumulate treasures in heaven, rather than on earth where rust and moth will destroy (Matthew 6:19-20).

## WHY DON'T WE EVER SEEM TO HAVE ENOUGH?

Because we spend money on things that do not satisfy the soul. However, there are things that money cannot buy; they are listed in Galatians:

> But the fruit of the Spirit is love, joy, peace,
> longsuffering, gentleness, goodness, faith, meekness,
> temperance: against such there is no law (5:22-23).

## WHY DO WE GET INTO DEBT TO ACQUIRE POSSESSIONS?

Again, it is a lack of trust, and not waiting on God to bless us. See, debt is not God's way for us to be blessed. The person in debt is a slave to the lender (Proverbs 22:7). Recognize where your complete source and resource comes from. Recognize that it is God who gives us the power to get wealth. Seek God's face and not His hands. "But seek ye first the kingdom of God, and his righteousness; and all these things shall be added unto you" (Matthew 6:33).

Forget about trying to impress others; if they do not accept you, oh well! As long as you are living according to God's standards and principals that are stated in the Bible, that is all that matters. Be a cheerful giver — to include your tithes and offerings. Give to those who are less fortunate.

Remember, God reserves true prosperity for His children. He will prosper us and allow us to succeed, according to Psalm 1:1-3 and Joshua 1:8. Material possession does not measure a person's value or spiritual merit!

*"But my God shall supply all your need*
*according to his riches in glory by Christ Jesus."*
-Philippians 4:19

SELF-CARE TIPS:

- What really matters to you?

- Be grateful for what you have.

- Show appreciation to others; give genuine compliments.

- The spiritual gifts and heart motivation, after all of the material possessions are gone, is what matters to God!

# NEGLECT

"...not forsaking the assembling of ourselves together,
as is the manner of some, but exhorting one another, and so
much the more as you see the Day approaching."
-Hebrews 10:25

ACCORDING TO THE DICTIONARY, NEGLECT MEANS "TO PAY little or no attention to; fail to heed; disregard: To fail to care for or attend to properly." Well, in this chapter, I am going to discuss the things we neglect. We have all experienced neglect in some shape, form, or fashion, whether we were the ones neglected, or we were the ones doing the neglecting. Worse yet, we neglect things that are important to God.

Personally, there have been times in the past when I felt neglected or left out, but here I will focus on what we neglect that are of utmost importance like health, finances, family, or the things of God.

I went through a period of neglecting all of the things that I just mentioned and ended up with a mess — a complete mess. In some strange way, I felt that if I ignored things (notices in the mail, bill collectors calling, negative balances in my checking and savings accounts), it would go away. We all know that is not true; I was a lot younger, not to mention my neglectful attitude toward God.

During this time, I also neglected my health, and by doing so, I jeopardized my health. I did not pay much attention to what I was eating, choosing to eat anything I wanted, and as much as I wanted. As a result, I developed hypertension, borderline diabetes, high cholesterol, and even kidney issues.

Also, you know what happens when you spend, spend, spend, or live without a budget — financial disaster, which is what happened to me before the national economic crisis hit. I was even advised to file for bankruptcy, but I did not, and thank God I did not.

And yes, I neglected God by not doing my reasonable service. How do we neglect God, you may be asking. We neglect God when we neglect the church and our responsibility to serve in it. We neglect God when we disobey Him. We neglect God when we go against sound biblical doctrine. We neglect God when we go against His will for our life. And, we neglect God when we disregard His teaching, as stated in Matthew 7:26: "And every one that heareth these sayings of mine, and doeth them not, shall be likened unto a foolish man, which built his house upon the sand."

I know, from personal experience, that God will turn your

life around. Whatever is lacking in your life, chances are, that is an area that you may have neglected.

SELF-CARE TIPS:

- Treat your body like the temple that it is. Remember, your health is not an occasion, but it is a lifestyle. Maintain a good healthy weight. Eat healthy and exercise regularly.

- If you are in debt, make a plan to get out. Develop a budget and stick to it. Tithe, save money, build financial wealth, and seek help from a financial planner if necessary. A little side note here, have multiple streams of income, so that you will always have money streaming in!

- Pray daily.

- Neglect not the gifts that He has given you.

- Last, but certainly not the least, make God first in your life. Read, study, worship, and obey His Word. Draw near to God, and He will draw closer to you.

# OPPORTUNITY

"Be wise in the way you act toward outsiders;
make the most of every opportunity."
-Colossians 4:5 NIV

EVERY DAY, WE ARE PRESENTED WITH A GIFT FROM GOD
that is full of opportunities. We are given another chance to
right our wrongs, mend our fences, bridge gaps, heal
relationships, and walk through the doors of opportunities that
God has for us. God reminds us in Revelation 3:8 that He has
set before us an open door that no one can shut; I don't know
about you, but that is a powerful promise.

God has already set an open door before us that no one can
shut, and you know God has wonderful gifts and promises for
us. Every good gift and every perfect gift is from above (James
1:17). So, that means that the open door is full of opportunities.

God also allows us to make choices; daily, He loads us with benefits and opportunities, and although it may not seem like it, opportunities will come — even though we may not always recognize them at first.

For example, not long after I moved to Georgia, I had a tough time finding a job. In fact, it was so bad, I could not even buy a job, and this was before the economic downturn. I searched high and low, sent resumes all over the place, had my resume professionally written and registered with at least five different employment agencies. *So, what was the problem?*

Again, this was way before the economic downturn of 2008. One day, by divine connection, I met a young lady at an intercessory prayer meeting and decided to ask her if she knew of any job opportunities. She said, "Yes, you can do what I do," and I said, "What is that?" She suggested that I sign up with a daycare employment agency.

I looked at her like she was crazy and started thinking in my mind: *Why would I want to work at a daycare?* Listen, I don't have any children myself, and I wasn't considering taking care of someone else's children. As a matter of fact, I thought this was one of the most ridiculous things I had heard in a while. I went on to say, "With my education and years of experience working for Corporate America, why in the world would I want to do that?" But this was the only door opening for me.

I took the information, thought about it for a few days, and then looked at my checkbook, which was on zero. I figured it was better to have something coming in than nothing, so I called the number, submitted all of my necessary credentials, completed a background check, and in less than a week, I was working, *you guessed it. . .* at a daycare.

My first assignment was to substitute for a few days at an exclusive private daycare. Now, this was all new to me; first, I had never heard of an agency for daycare teachers, and second, I had never heard of a private daycare for children. But we are in America, and anything is possible.

The few days turned into a few weeks, which turned into months, and eventually the whole school year. The children fell in love with me, and so did the parents and the school administration. It turned out to be a good fit for that season in my life, after all.

For Christmas that year, I received so many lovely gifts, cards, money, and more. So much so, that I had to make several trips to my car to carry it all out. I was also blessed with a bonus from the school. I felt so humbled that I cried because I was not expecting any of that. There is more —at the end of the school year, I got a job that was more in my chosen field. By this time, my assignment was over, and I was blessed with even more gifts and money.

This was the first time in my life that I cried when I left a job. Just look at what I would have missed had I not walked through that open door. Not to mention the joy that I received from teaching and training young, impressionable minds! So, as I stated earlier, opportunities are all around us. What may seem like an obstacle can actually turn out to be a great opportunity.

However, obstacles have a timeline, and God-given opportunities are for a lifetime; we may have to put in some hard work to recognize them, but they are there.

When opportunity knocks, and it will, embrace it with open arms. God has given you unlimited opportunities. The only person stopping you *is you*.

## SELF-CARE TIPS:

- Remember Revelation 3:8: "I know thy works: behold, I have set before thee an open door, and no man can shut it: for thou hast a little strength, and hast kept my word, and hast not denied my name."

- Meditate on Romans 8:28: "And we know that all things work together for good to them that love God, to them who are the called according to his purpose," and Jeremiah 29:11 (NIV): "For I know the plans I have for you, declares the LORD, plans to prosper you and not to harm you, plans to give you hope and a future."

- When faced with obstacles, remember you do have a choice. With God's help, you can turn that obstacle into a stepping stone to the promotion that God has for you. Take advantage of your opportunity.

- Use your creativity and imagination and stir up the gifts that God has given you.

- Exercise your faith. When faced with an obstacle, look at it as what it could be and not what it is.

# PRAYER

"Confess your trespasses to one another, and pray
for one another, that you may be healed. The effective, fervent
prayer of a righteous man avails much."

-James 5:16

THE WORD OF GOD ADMONISHES US TO PRAY WITHOUT
ceasing and is our direct line of communication with Him, so
prayer is the lifeblood for all Christians.

You have heard the saying, "prayer changes things," and it
does, but prayer changes us too. And, for Christians, prayer
should be our number one priority. We should pray for one
another, we should pray in faith, we should pray when things
are good, and we should pray when things are bad. We should
pray continually.

Prayer is a God-given priority, but we often use it to get

things from God, and it should also be used to develop a closer relationship with God.

Many of us pray when things are going well, and conversely, many of us only pray when things are chaotic. But we should always pray. Prayer is a tool that God gives to us to be more intimate with Him. Imagine if you did not communicate with your loved one, spouse, co-worker, friend, or anyone in your circle. How would you develop a relationship with them? The same is true of God; you must communicate with Him to develop a healthier relationship — this does not mean to talk to God only when you are in need, either. Prayer also provides us opportunities to praise Him, to thank Him, to petition Him, to repent to Him, and to intercede for others.

When we pray according to the will of God, circumstances change. I like to use the analogy of making a deposit in the bank. We save for emergencies, for future purchases; well, same here, there are times when things come at us so fast that we may not necessarily have time for long, deep prayer.

For example, once I was driving home from work on a busy highway in Maryland, when a truck traveling at a high rate of speed was headed right toward me. I just had enough time to scream out *Jee;* I did not even have enough time to call on the full name of Jesus. But God, in His grace, mercy, and protection, diverted that truck in the driver's proper lane. Whew! Thank you, Jesus!

Make prayer a priority and spend time with God in deep prayer so that you can make a withdrawal — when you need it.

There are times for deep prayers, but when a truck is headed toward you head-on, you need a quick one. Make prayer a priority.

Another example of how prayer can change or fix a situation or, in this case, healing, was when I was a child, I used to suffer from chronic bronchitis — which caused many trips to the hospital. On one particular occasion, I remember my Daddy sitting at the foot of my bed, praying.

In his prayer, I heard him say, "Lord Jesus, save my baby girl." Thank God I was healed, and thank God for a praying Daddy! James 5:16 says, "Confess your faults one to another, and pray one for another, that ye may be healed. The effectual fervent prayer of a righteous man avails much."

If you are not sure how to pray, or what to pray, my second book, *The Next Level,* has a chapter on praying, but I will briefly go over it again for those who may not be confident about how to pray. Prayer was a priority for Jesus as well. He prayed to His Father, and the disciples took note of this. The disciples also noticed how some of the priests at that time would stand in the synagogues, and on the street corners of the city so they could be seen.

But Jesus says when you pray, go into your room and shut the door and pray to your Father who will hear you in that secret place, and will reward you openly (Matthew 6:5-6). Also, Jesus gave us an example of how to pray in Matthew 6:8-13:

Be not ye therefore like unto them. For your Father

knoweth what things ye have need of, before ye ask
Him. After this manner therefore pray ye: Our Father
which art in heaven, Hallowed be thy name. Thy
kingdom come, thy will be done in earth, as it is in
heaven. Give us this day our daily bread. And forgive us
our debts, as we forgive our debtors. And lead us not
into temptation, but deliver us from evil: For thine is the
kingdom, and the power, and the glory, forever. Amen.

One last point that I want to drive home is knowing that
prayer is vital to everything you do. Pray for wisdom, pray for
knowledge, and pray to know God's will for your life.

Just pray!

## SELF-CARE TIPS:

- Pray from your heart; be honest in your prayer.

- Pray for yourself as well.

- Pray and meditate. Prayer is talking to God and
  meditation is listening to God.

- Pray with faith. James 5:14-16 says: "Is any sick
  among you? Let him call for the elders of the
  church; and let them pray over him, anointing him
  with oil in the name of the Lord: And the prayer of

faith shall save the sick, and the Lord shall raise him up; and if he have committed sins, they shall be forgiven him. Confess your faults one to another, and pray one for another, that ye may be healed. The effectual fervent prayer of a righteous man availeth much."

# QUITTING IS NOT AN OPTION

"And let us not be weary in well doing:
for in due season we shall reap, if we faint [quit] not."
-Galatians 6:9

BEGINNING THIS SECTION WITH THE ABOVE SCRIPTURE IS A
great start because it forewarns us that there may be times when
we will become weary, and may very well be tempted to quit.
However, it also admonishes us not to become so tired that we
give up, or give in, or give out; it holds a promise that we will
reap the benefits if we just don't faint. The Christian walk can
be challenging, yet rewarding.

The ways of the world are in stark contrast to the Word of
God. But, with the help of our Lord and Savior, we can do it.
This contrast creates constant friction between what the world
presents and what our Christian walk requires. We will have
trials and tribulations along the way.

That is one of the problems that I have with the "prosperity gospel". Some of its teaching is that everything will be a bed of roses, and this life will be trouble-free, but that is neither true nor scriptural. God clearly wants us to prosper in all that we do for Him, and He promises prosperity to His children, but we will face challenges, as well. But, when you come across these challenges — don't quit!

Many people today are faced with life's struggles, and the load seems to be a little too much to bear. When you overcome one thing, there is something else to conquer, lurking around the corner. Job had to deal with one thing after another, but he kept the faith. As a matter of fact, Job lost all of his earthly possessions, including his family, but he kept the faith. Job 13:15 says, "Though he slay me, yet will I trust in him: but I will maintain mine own ways before him."

So, hold on, your change is coming; your season will change, but don't quit. In fact, when the battle gets to be the hottest, that is usually a sign that your blessing, or breakthrough, is on the way. I've heard it said, "Your breakthrough comes just before your breakdown." See, if you quit, you will not fulfill the destiny that God has for you. God has great and mighty plans for each of us.

I went through a period when I was younger that I would just give up without putting forth much effort, dropping out of college toward the end of my junior year. At that point in time, I felt like I could not go on. The year and a half that I had left seemed like a lifetime, so I quit, moved to Washington, D.C., and got a job as a receptionist. I was pretty satisfied at first, but as time progressed, it was difficult for me to get promotions and move up the corporate ladder. Sure, I received accolades, but not having a college degree made it even more challenging.

So, I decided to go back to school part-time and finish the work to earn my degree. I have had many other obstacles in life since then, but I think about what would have happened if I quit. I am not like that now. I adopted the phrase "quitting is not an option," and you should, too.

Listen, wherever you are in life, if you have quit something, take a moment to consider whether it is something you can still go back to complete it. If it is, be prayerful about finishing it. What about that book that you started to write and did not finish? What about that college degree you always wanted? What about that business plan that you pushed to the wayside? What about any of the other projects that you quit? Pick it back up and complete it.

Sometimes, the only person in our way is ourselves. If you have failed at something. . . learn from the mistake and get back up and try it again. To encourage you to keep going and not quit, here is a list of a few individuals who kept going despite trials, tribulations, or delays. Some you may be familiar with, some are Old and New Testament saints, others are people from all walks of life:

- Albert Einstein was kicked out of school because of a lack of interest.
- Henry Ford (founder of Ford Motor Company) did not put a reverse gear in his first car.

- Abraham Lincoln lost nine elections before being elected President of the United States.
- Michael Jordon did not make the junior-varsity basketball team and was later told to join the military.
- Walt Disney went through adversity after adversity, but he kept going.
- Moses was a stutterer, but God used him to deliver the Hebrews out of Egypt.
- Joseph went from the pit to the palace.
- Esther was an orphan and later became a queen. Paul persecuted Christians, was transformed, and later wrote two-thirds of the books of the New Testament.

The Bible and many history books are replete with people that overcame adversity and were able to fulfill their God-ordained destiny. So, whatever it is that you are facing — don't quit. Do not let your age, color, education, or lack of (remember, you can always go back to school), disability, or whatever you are facing, cause you to quit. *Press on!*

Incidentally, God restored twice as much to Job than he had before (Job 42:10). Never, never, never, ever give up! Quitting is not an option.

*"I press toward the mark for the prize*
*of the high calling of God in Christ Jesus."*
-Philippians 3:14

SELF-CARE TIPS:

- There is so much more work to be done for the kingdom. There are souls to be saved, diseases that need cures, and new things waiting to be discovered.

- You may grow tired, you may get weary, but don't give up. Trust God for a bountiful harvest and the strength to keep on going.

- Exercise faith and patience to get to your destiny.

- God will complete His work, but you must be a willing vessel. Take a deep breath and keep moving forward.

# REST

"Take My yoke upon you and learn from Me,
for I am gentle and humble in heart, and you will find rest for
your souls. For my yoke is easy and My burden is light."
-Matthew 11:29-30

Come to me, all you who are weary
and burdened, and I will give you rest."
-Matthew 11:28 NIV

THE ALARM CLOCK GOES OFF, AND YOU BEGIN TO THINK about what the day has in store for you. You rush to get yourself dressed for the day, to cook breakfast for the family, and to get the kids ready for school. In some cases, many of you rush to help your spouse prepare for their day. Then, you rush off to work, only to find yourself stuck in traffic. Meanwhile, your smartphone or smartwatch is alerting you that you either have a text, email, phone call, or some other notification that demands your immediate attention.

After all of that, you rush through your work day, rush to get that report out, to eat lunch, and to get to that next meeting. Now, it is the end of the work day, but you are still in rush mode, as you are rushing to pick up the kids, get their dinner ready, and help with their homework. Rush, rush, rush. Did I mention after-school activities; such as soccer, piano lessons, dance lessons, or ministry meetings? Whew . . . this is enough to make you weary. Your to-do list has a to-do list. You are multitasking while multitasking. Incidentally, multitasking can short circuit your brain and reduce your performance and efficiency. When do you get a break?

Before I fully understood the power of resting, I used to rush and try to do everything. In some cases, my weekends were so busy that I even looked forward to the workweek - imagine that! It was not until one day, as I was rushing home to change clothes and grab a bite to eat, then to a meeting, when a powerful electrical storm came through and caused massive power outages.

Well, the power went out right about the time I was to leave the parking garage, which disabled the gate, so we could not exit. So, the only thing that I could do was rest and meditate. I was agitated, but what could I do? I interpreted that moment as a divine appointment with God, to stop and listen to what He had to say. The message was to slow down and rest.

You see, our Father God took time out to rest. Genesis 2:3 tells us that He rested on the seventh day from all of the work that He had done. Yes, God rested, so, if our Father in heaven took time to rest, so should we.

But I am here to tell you it is okay to rest. In fact, not only is it okay, it is necessary. Psalm 23:2-3 says:

> He maketh me to lie down in green pastures, He leads me beside the still waters. He restores my soul.

Rest in the Lord. Take some time right now and rest in Him. Close your eyes, inhale and exhale deeply and slowly, and imagine yourself crawling onto His lap and saying, "Abba Father, I need to rest in You right now." Try it! He will give you rest. Sometimes we just need to slow down and rest! Let this be your self-care. Don't feel guilty for enjoying some quiet time. Someone shared this example with me, and it goes something like this:

> When we are on an airplane, the flight attendant gives instructions that, in case of an emergency, we should put the oxygen mask on ourselves first, then proceed to assist those around us. In other words, self-care comes first; otherwise, we will be unable to help anyone else.

We are not Superwoman or Superman, nor are we robots, so at some point, if we don't slow down to rest, our bodies will break down to rest. God commands us to take a day and rest; it is one of the Ten Commandments: "Remember the Sabbath day, to keep it holy." (Exodus 20:8). Not only should we keep this day holy, but we should use it to meditate, rest, and relax. Taking a day to rest and relax will also help in alleviating stress and pressure.

SELF-CARE TIPS:

- Take time out to retreat, refresh, and rejuvenate your spirit and physical body.

- Meditate on Psalms 1:2-3: "But his delight is in the law of the LORD; and in his law doth he meditate day and night. And he shall be like a tree planted by the rivers of water, that bringeth forth his fruit in his season; his leaf also shall not wither; and whatsoever he doeth shall prosper."

- Carve out time for personal devotion to pray, read and study the Word of God — preferably early in the morning before your day starts.

- Listen to soft, soul-soothing music — praise and worship, jazz, or inspirational. "O sing unto the LORD a new song; for he hath done marvelous things: his right hand, and his holy arm, hath gotten him the victory." -Psalm 98:1

- Take a nice long walk in the park, one with

beautiful trees, luscious grass, and a sparkling lake. Enjoy nature. "He shall be like a tree planted by the rivers of water, that brings forth its fruit in its season, whose leaf also shall not wither; And whatever he does shall prosper." -Psalm 1:3

- Just rest and try doing nothing for a few hours for at least once a week.

# STRENGTH IN THE STORM

'

"But He said to them, "Where is your faith?"
And they were afraid, and marveled, saying to one another,
"Who can this be? For He commands even the winds
and water, and they obey Him!"
-Luke 8:25

SOMETIMES, WE REACH A POINT IN LIFE WHEN WE DON'T
know what to do; life has a tendency to zap our strength and
make us weary, worn out, and just plain weather-beaten. As
with natural storms, spiritual storms may, or may not, give us
warning signs that allow us to prepare ourselves ahead of time.
In either instance, these storms will most often have a
significant, and sometimes, long-lasting effect.

Even as I am writing this, our world, our country, is facing
an unprecedented and devastating pandemic. We are in the
middle of a plague that is reshaping our communities like never

before. Thousands have been stricken with this deadly virus, hundreds of thousands have died, and many have lost their jobs or sense of security. Life as we once knew it has changed. Our daily lives have been disrupted, the financial market has been rattled, and uncertainty abounds as anxiety and fear are at an all-time high. Entertainment, sports, schools have all been put on pause in an effort to flatten the curve.

Every day, we hear more devastating news than the day before. Is this a storm or what? In short, we are facing an economic and financial tsunami. But I am reminded that God says, "The righteous shall flourish like *the palm tree:* he shall grow like a cedar in Lebanon. Those that be planted in the house of the LORD shall flourish in the courts of our God" (Psalm 92: 12-13). This Scripture helps me to see that I had to stand firm during this time in our world. Let's take a look at that palm tree and learn from it, because it is designed to withstand hurricane-force winds.

Most tree roots get smaller and smaller the further down they go; however, the palm tree's roots are the same size at the base. This makes the tree difficult to uproot during a hurricane or bad storm. This also means the roots will grow deep into the ground, getting nourishment not available on the surface. Thus, David said a blessed man is "like a tree planted by the rivers of water that bringeth forth his fruit in his season" (Psalm 1:3).

God also commands us to "*take root downward, and bear fruit upward*" (Isaiah 37:31), which is precisely what the palm tree does. Another important fact about the palm tree is that most tree trunks are made up of dead wood, while the cambium layer (the living part of the tree) is just inside the bark. This makes it easy for animals to nibble around the bark at the bottom of the tree, thus killing it. The palm tree, on the other hand, has living wood throughout, making it harder to damage. This, coupled with the healthy root system and its flexibility, allows it to weather hurricane-force storms because it bends with the wind without breaking. When our lives are rooted in Christ (Col. 2:6-7), the storms of life will not break us. We may bend a little, but we will not break!

Fruit trees typically decrease in fruit production as they grow older. Palm trees do not bear fruit until they mature, which can take up to fifty years. But as the palm tree ages, the fruit grows sweeter. Yet, here is another promise of God: "They shall still bring forth fruit in old age; they shall be fat and flourishing" (Psalm 92:14 KJV). God does not want us to become fruitless in old age; our fruit should increase and become sweeter as the years pass.

And finally, the palm tree branch was a symbol of triumph and victory in both pre and early Christian times. The Romans rewarded champions of the games and celebrated military successes with palm branches. Early Christians used the palm branch to symbolize the victory of the faithful over their enemies, and the Palm Sunday festival celebrates the triumphal entry of Jesus into Jerusalem. In Judaism, the palm represents peace and plenty. In today's time, the palm tree still represents those very same things.

SELF-CARE TIPS:

- Remember the strength and makeup of the palm tree. Draw your strength from God during your season of adversity.

- Be rooted and grounded in the Word of God, so that you will be able to stand the winds and storms of life.

- Remember what Nehemiah 8:10b says, *"For the joy of the LORD is your strength."*

- Finally, remember in Mark 4:39 that Jesus rebuked the storm, and He can rebuke your storm, too. *"And He arose, and rebuked the wind, and said unto the sea, 'Peace, be still.' And the wind ceased, and there was a great calm."*

# TALENT, GIFTS, AND ABILITIES

"Every good gift and every perfect gift is from above,
and comes down from the Father of lights, with whom there is
no variation or shadow of turning."
-James 1:17

GOD HAS GIVEN EACH ONE OF US A TALENT OR GIFT AND, IN
many cases, both. Talents and gifts are very similar, yet different
in a specific kind of way. Both are from God, and both should be
shared with others; however, the primary difference is that
talent usually results from genetics, training, or exposure to a
particular environment; such as, sports or music. It is what God
gives us to make a living.

A gift, on the other hand, is given to all believers in Christ
by the Holy Spirit (Romans 12:6-8), to be used for the uplifting
of the kingdom and to bring God glory! Now that we have a
better understanding, we can move deeper into this message.

Many of us face a problem: We are not using our gift, talents, or abilities. This can be because of several reasons; one of which may be that some of us have been crushed at a young age because we were told that we couldn't sing, paint, or run as fast as someone else — or some other negative thing said to us. So, in many cases, we sit on our God-given gift. Some of us are fearful, but we must remember that God did not give us a spirit of fear, but of power, love, and a sound mind (2 Tim. 1:7). Whatever the case may be, we must push those things to the side and use our gifts to bring about a positive change in both our own, and someone else's, life.

About fifteen years ago, when I played the piano for the praise team, the church leader made a negative statement, because my style of playing was different from what he was accustomed to. Someone else heard that statement and pulled me to the side, reminding me that I can read music, but the individual criticizing me could not, and did not, know the difference between an A-flat and a G-sharp.

Unfortunately for me, I let that negativity get to me; it was years before I played any instrument again. So, don't let criticism stop you from using your God-ordained talents, gifts, or abilities. We have a responsibility to be a good steward over everything that God has given us, be it time, money, relationships, spouses, children, and our gifts, talents, and abilities. Those gifts will propel us into our destiny.

If we don't use what God has given us, we can lose it. I am reminded of the parables (story used to teach a lesson) in

Matthew 25:15-30; read it when you get an opportunity, but for now, I will summarize it for you.

A man needed his business to carry on while he was away on a long trip, so he gave one servant five talents, another servant was given two talents, and the other was given one. After returning, he summoned his servants, and this is what he found: The servant with the five talents and the servant with the two talents had each doubled their talents. But the servant that had one, complained and buried his talent.

The businessman took away the one talent that the servant had and gave it to the one who initially had five; the servant that previously had one talent, now had nothing — and was punished because of his decision not to use it.

The moral of this is, use whatever God has given you — use it wisely, and God will bless it and multiply it! By the way, I am skillfully playing my flute!

SELF-CARE TIPS:

- Discover your gifts and talents, if you haven't already.

- Perfect your gift, study your gift, and stir up your gifts.

- Use your spiritual gifts for kingdom building.

# UNITY

"Behold, how good and how pleasant it is
for brethren to dwell together in unity!"
-Psalms 133:1

BOY, DO WE NEED MORE OF THIS OR WHAT! I LOOKED UP
the definition of unity to make sure I had a clear understanding
of this word. Oddly enough, I found that singleness, integrity,
wholeness, and harmony were all synonyms for the word unity,
but the one that surprised me was integrity. But as I write this
piece, we will see how that comes into play.

Psalm 133:1 says, *"How good and pleasant it is when
brothers live together in unity."* Oh, how wonderful that would
be, if we would incorporate that Scripture into our daily lives.
We would probably finish so many projects on time; and think
about how much more effective our government, politicians,
churches, and organizations would be if we operate on that

principle. Yet, all too often, we are so busy bickering and jockeying for a high position, that we overlook the essential things.

Everyone wants to be the shining star, but no one wants to be in a supporting role; hence, this can cause division in our world. Working in unity also calls for a humble spirit. As I mentioned in a previous piece, to be promoted, we must first be humble. Luke 14:11 states, *"For whosoever exalteth himself shall be abased; and he that humbleth himself shall be exalted."*

The Book of Acts is replete with how the people came together on one accord (unity) to accomplish the work of the Lord. Acts 2:1-2 says:

> And when the day of Pentecost was fully come, they were all with one accord, in one place. And suddenly, there came a sound from heaven as of a rushing mighty wind, and it filled all the house where they were sitting. Because they were in unity, the Holy Spirit was able to perform miracles without dissention.

My musical background shows an example of how important it is to operate in unity. When the sopranos, altos, tenors, and bass singers and all of the musicians are on one accord, you have a beautiful choir that is singing to the glory of the Lord in harmony. But the minute someone is off-key or wants the spotlight on them, there is disharmony. We must all work together to accomplish one goal, and that is for kingdom building. We must put aside our own agenda and not focus on "me, myself, and I".

Disharmony and disunity can cause churches to divide, nations to fall, families to break up, and marriages to split. Disharmony is another tool of the enemy to keep us from walking in our preordained destiny. However, miracles can take place when all are on one accord. So, work in unity, place your focus on God, and remember why you are doing what you do.

SELF-CARE TIPS:

- Become one with Christ in unity and love.

- Remember there is no "I" in team. We all need our support system.

- Stay positive; for every singular negative thought, it takes three positive ones to counter it. Pause, breathe, and be grateful.

# VISION AND VICTORY

"Where there is no vision, the people perish:
but he that keepeth the law, happy is he."
-Proverbs 29:18

VISION AND VICTORY ARE TWO OF MY ABSOLUTE FAVORITE
topics. Many people go about life without realizing any true
purpose. Therefore, it can be difficult to face the day without
something positive to look forward to. It is my personal belief
that, many who suffer from certain forms of depression and
other life illnesses, do so because they have no sense of
direction, purpose, plan, or vision in their life; hence, they turn
to other things to cope.

I went through a period of searching for purpose in life
about seventeen years ago, so much so that I wrote a book
entitled "Answering the Call, Discovering Your Purpose." God

wants us to have a fulfilled life. He has the perfect plan for us, but we often miss it while in pursuit of other things.

I spent a lot of time praying, fasting, and seeking guidance for God's will in my life; and, I found it. You can also find yours by following the steps and instructions in this section, where you will learn how to write a mission and a vision statement — starting with Habakkuk 2:2-3:

> Then the Lord answered me and said: "Write the vision
> and make it plain on tablets, that he may run who reads
> it. For the vision is yet for an appointed time; but at the
> end it will speak, and it will not lie. Though it tarries,
> wait for it; Because it will surely come, It will not tarry.

That is a very powerful Scripture. The first thing it tells us to do is to write the vision. Your vision is for a set time (your season), and that, in the fullness of time, it will come to pass. Although it may not happen as quickly as you would like, it will happen. So, let's take a look at what mission and vision statements are.

## MISSION STATEMENT

A mission statement is an expression of what you stand for, of what you believe. It reflects your character, your accountability, your responsibility, your intended goals, your commitment, and your actions. In essence, it is a fundamental, or foundational, statement of your standards and plan of action.

A mission statement should be your personal constitution. It should include your ministry, your family, your health, and your finances.

## VISION STATEMENT

Now, what is a vision statement? Or, better yet, what is your personal vision? It is a look into a future filled with God's promises for your life. It is the ability to anticipate, visualize, or foresee an expected plan for your future, and the development of a course of action that moves you along destiny's course.

Vision serves as pictorial enlightenment of who you are and what you are moving toward. It's what lights your way as you journey (by faith) toward the destination that God has in store for you.[1] In simpler terms, vision is your GPS.

Together, your mission statement and vision statement are tools that will assist you in walking into your destiny.

## GUIDELINES FOR WRITING A MISSION STATEMENT

- It must be flexible. It must be inspiring.
- It must benefit one person or party/group. It must make sense.
- It is not a to-do list.
- It should be operable 24/7 (in other words, if you were to wake up in the middle of the night, you can still live by your mission statement).

## GUIDELINES FOR WRITING A VISION STATEMENT

- Write one important goal for each following item: physical, spiritual, work or career, family, social relationships, financial security, and fun.
- List three things you must do every day to feel fulfilled in your life and work.
- What would you do for free? What would you regret not doing?
- Your vision statement should be no more than thirty words.

## VISION BOARD

One more component for this is a vision board. A vision board is a tool used to help clarify, concentrate, and maintain focus on a specific life goal; it is any sort of board on which you display images that represent whatever you want to be, do, or have in your life.[2] A vision board helps to:

- Identify your vision and gives it clarity. Reaffirms your daily affirmations.
- It helps you to stay focused. Be specific on what you want.
- Your vision board can be text, or pictures, or both (mine is both).
- Your vision board should include what you want

your finances to be, your relationship, your health, and of course, your walk with God.

Tools needed to create your vision board: Poster board, scissors, glue stick, magazine or newspaper, and your creativity.

SELF-CARE TIPS:

- Follow the instructions in Habakkuk 2:2-3.

- Write both a mission *and* a vision statement.

- Create a vision board and place it where you can see it first thing in the morning; view it regularly.

- Consult with a life coach to keep you on track!

## WHAT, WHERE, WHEN, WHY, AND HOW, LORD?

"How long, O Lord? Will You forget me forever?
How long will You hide Your face from me?
How long shall I take counsel in my soul,
*Having* sorrow in my heart daily?
How long will my enemy be exalted over me?
Consider *and* hear me, O Lord my God;
Enlighten my eyes, Lest I sleep the *sleep of* death;
Lest my enemy say, "I have prevailed against him";
*Lest* those who trouble me rejoice when I am moved.
But I have trusted in Your mercy;
My heart shall rejoice in Your salvation.
I will sing to the Lord,
Because He has dealt bountifully with me."

-Psalm 13:1-6 NKJV

WE ALL GO THROUGH DIFFICULT TIMES IN OUR LIVES WHEN events that happen do not make any sense — that is what this book is all about; its purpose is to help you navigate those times. We want to question God about what is going on with us. Many of us have been taught that it is improper to question God; however, I disagree with that teaching. God gave us a reasoning mind (no, we will not have the answer to everything), and He already knows what is going on in our head anyway.

How many times are we faced with situations when we cry out: "Lord, I am your child. I go to church every Sunday and Bible study during the week, I pay my tithes, I treat everybody right, and I read and study my Bible. Why is this happening to me"? Well, let me just say this to you, *don't get weary*. You cannot go wrong by doing right.

Getting tired or fatigued is physical, but weary is spiritual. God promises to satisfy the weary and replenish the sorrowful heart: "For I have satiated the weary soul, and I have replenished every sorrowful soul" (Jeremiah 31:25).

Let's take a look at some of the Old and New Testament saints in the Bible. Moses certainly questioned God from time to time. Thomas had his doubts. Job had his debates with God, and Jesus, His own son, cried out with questions. So, it only stands to reason that we will have questions, too.

In this writing, I want to focus on a little-known prophet named Habakkuk. Not much is known about him, other than he was a prophet (God's mouthpiece), and was not afraid to ask questions about things he did not understand. He lived in a time when there was a lot of injustice, and a lack of integrity, selfishness, and lawlessness among God's people. Sounds like now, right? Still, the key phrase here is these were God's people — believers.

Habakkuk was complaining and praising God, all in the same breath (sounds like me from time to time). He did not understand why God was not moving quick enough to stop the behavior of the people; and to top that off, God was going to use the Babylonians, *their enemies*, to bring about their punishment. Habakkuk was very upset, so he cried out, "Why, Lord? How long, Lord?" (Habakkuk 1:1-4).

God may not necessarily answer our questions right away, but He will in His time and in His way. We must remember that God knows the plans He has for us; He knows our future. We must trust Him in every aspect of our daily life. And yes, God did answer Habakkuk. He gave Him detailed instructions:

> I will stand upon my watch, and set me upon the tower, and will watch to see what he will say unto me, and what I shall answer when I am reproved. And the Lord answered me, and said, Write the vision, and make it plain upon tables, that he may run that readeth it. For the vision is yet for an appointed time, but at the end it shall speak, and not lie: though it tarry, wait for it; because it will surely come, it will not tarry.
>
> -Habakkuk 2:1-3

SELF-CARE TIPS:

- Continue your course, as long as you are living right and holy, according to the Word of God.

- Create your own self-care plan; one that works best for you and includes the following: *Physical* self-care, *Social* self-care, *Mental* self-care, and *Spiritual* self-care.

- God will complete what He has started in you, even though we will have trials and tribulations, as long as we are doing a reasonable service.

# E(X)AMINE YOURSELF

"Let us search out and examine
our ways, and turn back to the Lord . . ."
-Lamentations 3:40

WE OFTEN HEAR THE TERM "IT'S NOT ABOUT YOU,"
especially in the Christian arena, and in some cases, that is true;
however, in many cases, we do need to focus on ourselves. The
word of God says, "Let a man examine himself." There are
things we do need to look at deep down in our souls, especially
when we find fault with another person. Matthew 7:2-4 says:

> For with what judgment you judge, you will be judged;
> and with the measure you use, it will be measured back
> to you. And why do you look at the speck in your
> brother's eye, but do not consider the plank in your own

eye? Or how can you say to your brother, 'Let me remove the speck from your eye'; and look, a plank is in your own eye?

Before we criticize or disapprove of another person's actions, consider the situation that you are in. How many times do we say, "If I were her, I would do this", or "She should do this", or "He would be better off if he does such and such?" We are quick to analyze someone else's personal affairs – how someone else should spend their money, how they should raise their children, where they should live or work, and how they should handle their relationships, and even to the point of where someone else should attend church.

Yes, we do need to pray and offer suggestions so that person can make wise decisions, but sometimes we can go overboard, which becomes judgmental rather than helpful! Which brings us to motivation. *Why* do we do the things we do? Someone may give a large sum of money to a church, or organization to earn a tax break, while others may give from their heart because of the compassion they may have for the less fortunate. Then, there are those whose purpose is to receive praise and attention.

What is your motivation? The sixth chapter of Matthew warns us to be careful of our charitable deeds — not to be seen by others when we give; if we give in secret, God will reward us openly. It goes a little further regarding prayer and fasting. Some of the 'hypocrites' of that time loved to be seen praying on the corners of the street. Yes, we should pray, but we should not do it just to be seen. Also, with fasting, we should not appear, or appeal, to man but unto our Father (needs clarity) — if we do this in secret, He will reward us openly.

Again, my question is, what is your motive? Examine yourself. We should be moved by our hearts and not by selfishness, or to gain attention. You want your "offering" to be accepted by God because His reward is the best.

A few years ago, I worked with a lady who often fasted for spiritual reasons. But it was a complete turnoff to everyone who was around her during this time. She constantly complained about having a headache or stomachache. Heaven forbid we happened to have a luncheon during her time of fasting; she would always say it was the devil that did not want her to fast. Yet, others would be on a fast, and you never knew until it was over. There were times I would fast and would carry on as usual — meaning, I did not announce that I was fasting, and when it came to the working lunch, I would just say, "Not today."

SELF-CARE TIPS:

- When you are doing a task, remember to do it unto the Lord, and not to be seen for vainglory.

- Focus on activities that you enjoy.

- Take breaks for your electronic devices and social media.

- God is the only one who truly knows your heart. Ask Him to reveal any area of your heart that needs to be purified. Ask God to order and direct your steps.

# YIELD

"Be not deceived; God is not mocked:
for whatsoever a man soweth, that shall he also reap."
-Galatians 6:7

I received a notice in the mail, stating something to the effect that my renewal interest rate and annual percentage *yield* would be available on a specified date, and could be obtained by contacting my financial center. We hear the word *yield* from time to time, especially in the financial arena and in the Bible. So, what does it mean?

Yield means *to give a return, as for labor expended; produce; bear.*

Oftentimes, we spin our wheels going nowhere fast, without yielding any results, or at least the results we hope for. It's the equivalent of being on a treadmill expending energy, but not going anywhere.

You may be asking yourself, '*Why am I not yielding the results I had forecasted?*' Or, '*Why aren't my dreams coming to pass; it seems for every one step that I take, I feel like I have been pushed back three.*'

Once I had written a couple of books, I realized that there was a lot more work involved than I had ever anticipated. With my first book, the sales were very soft, and I had to rethink, and even get help, especially with marketing. Now I have a better handle on what to do to increase my sales—good publishers, marketing, public relations, and media are all needed to get my yield.

The Bible says in Galatians 6:7 that "we are not to be deceived. That God is not mocked, and that whatever a man sows, that he will also reap." In other words, if you plant carrots, don't expect to yield apples — a simple, yet profound example. Maybe, just maybe, we are producing from a bad crop of seeds that we have planted. Alright, so what do we do now? Let's pull up those undesired results and start over the right way.

Decide what you want to yield. Then, count the cost before you start your project — be it to start a business, or your own radio, television, or ministry. It is crucial to know what you will need in terms of finances, staff, patents, lawyer, accountant, tax account, marketing, advertising, and so on. The average person, yielding their desired results, did not just wake up one morning and start a project without giving thought to it; a lot of time, energy, and effort went into it.

If you are interested in having a television or radio program, YouTube channel, or podcast, do the necessary work to find out what is expected. Take a tour of a radio or TV station to get a better understanding of what is involved. Consider shadowing a person who is where you would like to be and learn from them.

Again, for emphasis, check out what you are sowing. For love, sow love, for joy, sow joy. If you want to be blessed, give; if you want wealth, invest wisely, and save. If you want honor, live honorably; if you want an education, 'study to show thyself approved'. And, if you want to be physically fit, exercise and eat healthy. Conversely, if you borrow money, you could end up in debt; if you sow seeds of discord, you could yield a life of misery, and if you eat food loaded with high fat, sugar and calories — and couple that with lack of exercise — you will probably yield an unhealthy lifestyle. Also, if you do nothing, you will yield nothing. In the same vein, we reap the proportion of what we sow. Remember this:

"Whoever sows sparingly will also reap sparingly,
and whoever sows generously will also reap generously."
-2 Corinthians 9:6

SELF- CARE TIPS

- If you are not yielding the results that you are striving for, ask the Master to help you plant good seeds. Fertilize your seed with God's Word, water it

JENNIFER STOVALL EICHELBERGER

daily with the Holy Spirit, and continue to nourish it with faith. It is God who gives the increase.

- Keep in mind that we yield in a different season than we sow. "Even as I have seen, those who plow iniquity, and sow trouble reap the same" -Job 4:8

- Speak positive thoughts to yourself.

# ZERO

"Bearing with one another, and forgiving one another, if anyone has a complaint against another; even as Christ forgave you, so you also *must do*. But above all these things put on love, which is the bond of perfection. And let the peace of God rule in your hearts, to which also you were called in one body; and be thankful. Let the word of Christ dwell in you richly in all wisdom, teaching and admonishing one another in psalms and hymns and spiritual songs, singing with grace in your hearts to the Lord. And whatever you do in word or deed, *do* all in the name of the Lord Jesus, giving thanks to God the Father through Him."

-Colossians 3:13-23

ZERO IS WHEN SOMETHING HAS REACHED ITS LOWEST point, or the point of exhaustion, as in "my tolerance level is zero", or "I have zero degrees of patience with someone or something." When placed in the front of a number, zero can diminish the value, but when placed behind a number, it can significantly increase its value; for example: 1, 10, 100, 1,000, 10,000 to one million and beyond.

However, as Christ followers, we are exposed to many non-Christlike things; we are often placed in circumstances where we either tolerate it or we don't. A prime example is traveling on a subway, or an airplane when there are back-ups or delays, and tempers are flaring. These types of situations can often bring out the worst in people. You may hear foul language, or even witness obnoxious behavior. You can either try to ignore it as much as you can, pray for peace, or exercise your 'holy boldness' and speak up.

Frankly, I opt to pray for peace. Even in Corporate America, we are somewhat forced to be tolerant of all kinds of things, and if we are not, we are required to attend a sensitivity training program. We are living in a society where just about anything goes, our tolerance level hitting zero for most of us. As Christians, we are labeled, or persecuted, if we stand up for our belief, but yet, this "worldly tolerance" is pushed down our throats. Many of us verbalize our zero tolerance on other people, but as stated above, some things we can avoid, some things we can't, and some things we should.

Zero tolerance is very personal to me. There have been many times when I have fallen short, but because of His love, grace, mercy, and longsuffering, God is tolerant of me! The next time you come across something, or more than likely, someone that you have zero tolerance for— remember God's grace and mercy that He has for you.

Yes, there are some things we should have zero tolerance for as Christians, and some of them are mentioned in Galatians 5:19-21:

> Now the works of the flesh are manifest, which are these; adultery, fornication, uncleanness, lasciviousness, idolatry, witchcraft, hatred, variance, emulations, wrath, strife, seditions, heresies, envyings, murders, drunkenness, revelings, and such like: of the which I tell you before, as I have also told you in time past, that they which do such things shall not inherit the kingdom of God.

Still, we should exercise love, patience, and of course, pray for those individuals. Remember, you 'can do all things through Christ who strengthens' you!

## SELF-CARE TIPS:

- Love: The source of God is love. "And this is His commandment, that we should believe on the name of His Son Jesus Christ, and love one another, as He gave us commandment." -1 John 3:23

- Joy: "Then he said unto them, Go your way, eat the fat, and drink the sweet, and send portions unto them for whom nothing is prepared: for this day is holy unto our LORD: neither be ye sorry; for the joy of the LORD is your strength." -Nehemiah 8:10

- Peace: "And the peace of God, which passeth all understanding, shall keep your hearts and minds through Christ Jesus."- Philippians 4:7

- Patience: "But let patience have her perfect work, that ye may be perfect and entire, wanting nothing." -James 1:4

- Kindness: "Put on therefore, as the elect of God, holy and beloved, bowels of mercies, kindness, humbleness of mind, meekness, longsuffering." - Colossians 3:12

- Goodness: "A good man out of the good treasure of the heart bringeth forth good things: and an evil man out of the evil treasure bringeth forth evil things." -Matthew 12:35

- Faithfulness: "He that is faithful in that which is least is faithful also in much: and he that is unjust in the least is unjust also in much." -Luke 16:10

- Gentleness: "And the servant of the Lord must not strive; but be gentle unto all men, apt to teach, patient..." -2 Timothy 2:24

- Self-control: "And beside this, giving all diligence, add to your faith virtue; and to virtue knowledge; and to knowledge temperance; and to temperance patience; and to patience godliness." -2 Peter 1:5-6

# CONCLUSION

*Thank you* for taking this journey with me, and I pray that this book has been a blessing to you, especially in terms of self-care. I wrote this book in hopes of helping you, if —and when — you experience some of the things that I have experienced.

Remember that self-care is not selfish. It is imperative to implement the steps outlined in this book to help you maintain your health and well-being. Based on the tools and tips in the book, develop a plan of self-care, making sure to include activities you enjoy. Put this plan in a place where you can easily see it, and practice these activities daily. The following sections include additional personal tips and Scriptures to support you on your self-care journey.

Be well!

# ADDITIONAL SELF-CARE TIPS

- Pray and meditate about everything.
- Learn and practice the proper techniques for breathing.
- Read a good book; start with the Bible.
- Spend time in nature; enjoy the beach, the sun, and the grass.
- Do something creative: cook, learn to play an instrument, take an art class, learn a new language. Start a bucket list.
- Travel.
- Read inspirational quotes.
- Treat yourself to comfort food from time to time. Enjoy an ice cream cone.
- Organize your living space. Create a creative room.
- Listen to jazz or soothing music.

- Develop your own self-care techniques. Start your day with prayer.
- Forgive yourself. Drink plenty of water.
- Take a new route to work.
- Move your body; exercise, dance. Detox from negativity.
- Decompress throughout the day; such as, deep breathing and meditating.
- Get plenty of rest and sleep.
- Treat yourself with love, kindness, and compassion. Love yourself and others unconditionally.
- Journal.
- Practice gratitude. Have a digital detox. Buy fresh flowers.
- Volunteer to help others. Speak positive thoughts.
- Remember, self-care isn't selfish.

# SUPPORT SCRIPTURES

Someone reading this book could be dealing with some severe and immediate concerns, but we know that God is able! Meditate on the following Scriptures for your needs!

## HEALING:

"I shall not die, but live, and declare the works of the LORD."

-Psalms 118:17

"But He was wounded for our transgressions, He was bruised for our iniquities; the chastisement for our peace was upon Him, and by His stripes we are healed."

-Isaiah 53:5

"Now when Jesus had come into Peter's house, He saw his wife's mother, lying sick with a fever. So, He touched her hand, and the fever left her. And she arose and served them.

When evening had come, they brought to Him many who were demon-possessed. And He cast out the spirits with a word, and healed all who were sick, that it might be fulfilled, which was spoken by Isaiah the prophet..."

-Matthew 8:14-17

"Who forgives all your iniquities, who heals all your diseases, who redeems your life from destruction, who crowns you with lovingkindness and tender mercies, who satisfies your mouth with good things, so that your youth is renewed like the eagle's."

-Psalms 103:3-5

"Who Himself bore our sins in His own body on the tree, that we, having died to sins, might live for righteousness—by whose stripes you were healed."

-1 Peter 2:24

GRATITUDE:

"Let everything that hath breath praise the LORD. Praise ye the LORD."

-Psalms 150:6

SUFFICIENCY:

"Do not lay up for yourselves treasures on earth, where moth and rust destroy and where thieves break in and steal; but lay up for yourselves treasures in heaven, where neither moth nor rust destroys and where thieves do not break in and steal. For where your treasure is, there your heart will be also."

-Matthew 6:19-21

"And let us not be weary in well doing: for in due season we shall reap, if we faint not."

-Galatians 6:9

"This Book of the Law shall not depart from your mouth, but you shall meditate in it day and night, that you may observe to do according to all that is written in it. For then you will make your way prosperous, and then you will have good success."

-Joshua 1:8

"Being confident of this very thing, that he which hath begun a good work in you will perform it until the day of Jesus Christ."

-Philippians 1:6

"For I know the thoughts that I think toward you, saith the LORD, thoughts of peace, and not of evil, to give you an expected end."

-Jeremiah 29:11

REST:

"Come to Me, all you who labor and are heavy laden, and I will give you rest."

-Matthew 11:28

"And He said to them, "Come aside by yourselves to a deserted place and rest a while." For there were many coming and going, and they did not even have time to eat."

-Mark 6:31

"Be still, and know that I am God: I will be exalted among the heathen, I will be exalted in the earth."

-Psalms 46:10

GIFTS:

"And God hath set some in the church, first apostles, secondarily prophets, thirdly teachers, after that miracles, then gifts of healings, helps, governments, diversities of tongues. Are all apostles? Are all prophets? Are all teachers? Are all workers of miracles? Have all the gifts of healing? Do all speak with tongues? Do all interpret? But covet earnestly the best gifts: and yet shew I unto you a more excellent way."

-1 Corinthians 12:27-31

"And he gave some, apostles; and some, prophets; and some, evangelists; and some, pastors and teachers; For the perfecting of the saints, for the work of the ministry, for the edifying of the body of Christ."

-Ephesians 4: 11-12

"Therefore, I remind you to stir up the gift of God, which is in you through the laying on of my hands."

-2 Timothy 1:6

"Neglect not the gift that is in thee, which was given thee by prophecy, with the laying on of the hands of the presbytery."

-1 Timothy 4:14

"Every good gift and every perfect gift is from above, and cometh down from the Father of lights, with whom is no variableness, neither shadow of turning."

- James 1:17

"There are diversities of gifts, but the same Spirit. And there are differences of administrations, but the same Lord. And there are diversities of operations, but it is the same God which worketh all in all. But the manifestation of the Spirit is given to every man to profit withal."

-1 Corinthians 12: 4-7

UNITY:

"And the people with one accord gave heed unto those things which Philip spake, hearing and seeing the miracles which he did."

-Acts 8:6

"And by the hands of the apostles were many signs and wonders wrought among the people; (and they were all with one accord in Solomon's porch.)."

-Acts 5:12

"Fulfill ye my joy, that ye be like-minded, having the same love, being of one accord, of one mind."

-Philippians 2:2

STRENGTH:

"He giveth power to the faint; and to them that have no might, he increaseth strength. Even the youths shall faint and be weary, and the young men shall utterly fall: But they that wait upon the LORD shall renew their strength; they shall mount up with wings as eagles; they shall run, and not be weary; and they shall walk, and not faint."

-Isaiah 40:29-31

"Fret not thyself because of evildoers, neither be thou envious against the workers of iniquity. For they shall soon be cut down like the grass, and wither as the green herb.

Trust in the LORD, and do good; so shalt thou dwell in the land, and verily thou shalt be fed. Delight thyself also in the LORD: and he shall give thee the desires of thine heart. Commit thy way unto the LORD; trust also in him; and he shall bring it to pass."

-Psalm 37:1-5

"Being confident of this very thing, that he which hath begun a good work in you will perform it until the day of Jesus Christ."

-Philippians 1:6

"I press toward the mark for the prize of the high calling of God in Christ Jesus."

-Philippians 3:14

EXAMINE YOURSELF:

"Search me, O God, and know my heart: try me, and know my thoughts: And see if there be any wicked way in me, and lead me in the way everlasting."

-Psalm 139:23-24

"Every way of a man is right in his own eyes: but the LORD ponders the hearts."

-Proverbs 21:2

"Create in me a clean heart, O God; and renew a right spirit within me."

-Psalm 51:10

"Take heed that you do not do your charitable deeds before men, to be seen by them. Otherwise, you have no reward from your Father in heaven. Therefore, when you do a charitable deed, do not sound a trumpet before you as the hypocrites do in the synagogues and in the streets, that they may have glory from men. Assuredly, I say to you, they have their reward.

But when you do a charitable deed, do not let your left hand know what your right hand is doing, that your charitable deed may be in secret; and your Father, who sees in secret will Himself reward you openly."

-Matthew 6: 1-4

"Let a man so consider us, as servants of Christ and stewards of the mysteries of God. Moreover, it is required in stewards that one be found faithful. But with me, it is a very small thing that I should be judged by you or by a human court. In fact, I do not even judge myself. For I know of nothing against myself, yet I am not justified by this; but He who judges me is the Lord.

Therefore, judge nothing before the time, until the Lord comes, who will both bring to light the hidden things of darkness and reveal the counsels of the heart. Then each one's praise will come from God."

-1 Corinthians 4:1-5

## SOWING:

"Who then is Paul, and who is Apollos, but ministers by whom ye believed, even as the Lord gave to every man? I have planted, Apollos watered; but God gave the increase. So then neither is he that planteth anything, neither he that watereth; but God that giveth the increase.

Now he that planteth and he that watereth are one: and every man shall receive his own reward according to his own labour. For we are labourers together with God: ye are God's husbandry, ye are God's building."

-1 Corinthians 3:5-9

"To everything there is a season, a time for every purpose under heaven."

-Ecclesiastes 3:1

"You will know them by their fruits. Do men gather grapes from thorn bushes or figs from thistles? Even so, every good tree bears good fruit, but a bad tree bears bad fruit."

-Matthew 7:16-17

# NOTES

## VISION AND VICTORY

1. https://blog.mindvalley.com/vision-board/
2. https://stepintosuccessnow.com/

# ABOUT THE AUTHOR

Rev. Dr. Jennifer Stovall Eichelberger has an extensive background in Christian radio and television production and programming. Appearing, producing, and hosting shows focused on women in ministry, such as "Essence of Grace" and "Christian Women in Mass Media." She also produced and co-hosted "Sound Doctrine," a radio program featuring Christian artists and writers.

She is the former senior producer of WATC TV-57's "Atlanta Live" flagship show, and she has also produced many other programs, including cooking shows and fitness segments, emphasizing healthy eating habits and gospel music shows. Rev. Jennifer has recently been named senior producer and program manager at Inspiration Television Network (ITN).

She resides in the metropolitan Atlanta area with her husband, the legendary Dr. Herbert Lewis Eichelberger, a world-renowned professor and film director.

Learn more about Jennifer and her ministry at:
www.jennifereichelberger.com

Made in USA - North Chelmsford, MA
77543_9781734963700
02.23.2024 1307